HOW TO USE BICARBONATE

A Complete Step-By-Step Guide On How Baking Soda Treats Various Health Conditions, Prevents Kidney Diseases, Applies To Pets, And Boosts Exercise Performance

By

Dr. Grayson Owen

Copyright@2023

Table of Contents

CHAPTER ONE 12

  INTRODUCTION..........................12

    What is baking soda? 14

    Health challenges where healing with baking soda is effective........15

    Pros and cons of healing with baking soda..................................15

    Myths surrounding the uses of baking soda..................................17

    Benefits of using baking soda 18

CHAPTER TWO 19

  HISTORY OF SODIUM BICARBONATE 19

    Ancient use of alkaline substances era..19

    The scientific understanding era ..20

    Leavening in the baking era 20

    The commercial production era ...21

    The medicinal use 21

    The widespread usage era 22

    The diverse applications era.........23

    In contemporary times..................23

CHAPTER THREE 25
THE CHEMISTRY OF SODIUM BICARBONATE 25
Chemical structure 25
    Bicarbonate ion 25
    Acid-base properties 26
    Reaction with acids 27
    Leavening action in baking 27
    Decomposition at high temperatures 28
    Alkalinity and pH regulation 28
Sources 29
    Natural deposits 29
    Synthetic production 29
    Chemical industries 30
    Mining and extraction 30
    Commercial suppliers 31
    Retail stores 31
Extraction Methods 31
    Mining from natural deposits 31
    Solution mining 32
    Solvay process 33

Reaction with carbon dioxide.......33
  Neutralization reaction 33
  Electrolysis...................................34
  Purification and crystallization 35
Grades 35
  Food grade....................................35
  Pharmaceutical grade 37
  United States Pharmacopeia grade
 37
  Technical grade 38
  Industrial grade............................39
  Agricultural grade 40
  Reagent grade..............................40
  Cosmetic grade............................41
  Specialty grades 42
Properties..42
  Physical properties 42
  Chemical properties 44
Laboratory preparation.....................46
  Using sodium carbonate and carbon dioxide..46
The commercial production 47

Raw materials 47
First step: formation of sodium bicarbonate 48
Second step: regeneration of ammonium chloride 49
Third step: recovery of sodium carbonate 49

CHAPTER FOUR 51

HEALING ACTIONS AND PROPERTIES 51
Antacid properties 51
Abrasive properties 51
Anti-inflammatory and soothing properties 52
Antifungal and odor-neutralizing properties 53
Alkaline properties 53
Alkalization properties 54
Buffering capacity 55

CHAPTER FIVE 56

DEVICES FOR USE WITH SODIUM BICARBONATE 56
Devices and methods 56

Nebulizers 56

Dental applications 64

Using a toothbrush for oral hygiene 64

Infusion pumps for urinary alkalinization 67

Skin and scalp applicators 70

Sprayers for Oral conditions 72

CHAPTER SIX 75

FORMS BAKING SODA CAN BE CONSUMED 75

Baking soda solution 75

Baking soda paste 76

Cooking and baking 77

Oral rinse 79

Toothpaste 80

Antacid tablets 81

Supplements 82

Beverage additive 83

Dissolved in juice 84

CHAPTER SEVEN 85

PRECAUTIONS 85

    Consulting healthcare professional 85

    Dosage and administration 87

    Avoid prolonged use 89

    Monitor sodium levels.................. 91

    Dental precautions........................ 92

    Respiratory precautions................ 93

    Adverse reactions 95

    Child safety 97

    Storing safely 100

    Educating oneself 102

    Follow professional advice 104

CHAPTER EIGHT............................ 107

APPLICATION TO VARIOUS CONDITIONS 107

    What is heartburn? 107

    Causes of heartburn 107

    Symptoms of heartburn 108

    How can you use baking soda to relief heartburn? 108

    What is indigestion? 109

    Causes of indigestion 109

- Symptoms of indigestion............110
- How can you use baking soda to relieve indigestion? 110

What is metabolic acidosis? 112
- Causes metabolic acidosis..........112
- Symptoms metabolic acidosis 112
- How can you use baking soda to relieve metabolic acidosis? 113

What is dental plaque? 113
- Causes of dental plaque..............113
- Symptoms of dental plaque 114
- How can you use baking soda to treat dental plaque? 114

What is eczema?..............................115
- Causes of eczema 115
- Symptoms of eczema 115
- How can you use baking soda to relieve eczema symptoms?..........117

What is foot odor? 118
- Causes of foot odor 118
- Symptoms of foot odor...............119
- How can you use baking soda to manage foot odor........................119

What are mouth ulcers?...................120

    Causes of mouth ulcers 120

    Symptoms of mouth ulcers.........120

    How can you use baking soda to alleviate mouth ulcers?...............120

What is sunburned skin? 121

    Causes of sunburned skin...........121

    Symptoms of sunburned skin 121

    How can you use baking soda to offer relief for sunburn skin?.......121

What are chemical burns? 122

    Causes of chemical burns...........122

    Symptoms of chemical burns 122

    How can you use baking soda to provide relief to chemical burns? 123

What are insect bites or stings?......124

    Causes of insect bites or stings...124

    Symptoms of insect bites or stings 125

    How can you use baking soda to provide relief to insect bites or stings?..125

What is a poison oak rash?.............126

   Causes of poison oak rash..........127

   Symptoms of poison oak rash....127

   How can you use baking soda to provide relief to poison oak rash?...128

What is optimal exercise performance?..................................129

   Factors affecting exercise performance................................129

   Symptoms of optimal exercise performance................................129

   How can you use baking soda to boost exercise performance?......130

What are kidney diseases? 131

   Causes of kidney diseases..........131

   Symptoms of kidney diseases....132

   How can you use baking soda to prevent kidney diseases?............133

Baking soda and pets......................134

   Uses and considerations for pets 134

   What is oral hygiene for pets?....135

How can you use baking soda for oral hygiene in pets?................135

What is odor in pet's bedding? 136

How can you use baking soda to control the odor in your pet's bedding? 136

What are the itching and discomfort from insect bites and stings in pets? 137

Symptoms..................................137

How can you use baking soda to offer relief for it in pets? 138

CHAPTER NINE 139

CONCLUSIONS............................139

Index..141

CHAPTER ONE

INTRODUCTION

Do you seek a book with an in-depth guide to know how sodium bicarbonate functions and how to use it to relieve heartburn, indigestion, chemical burn, itching, inflammation from insect bites or stings, treat dental plaque, eczema, some health issues in pets, prevent kidney damage, optimize exercise performance, and several other health challenges with ease? Seek no further, as this is the most excellent book to study, comprehend, and be well-informed to help alleviate all these ailments. It is a guide for individuals who seek to accomplish exceptional outcomes. Several illustrations have also been added for your comprehension.

The objectives of this book include, first, highlighting the complete, step-by-step guide on how baking soda treats different health conditions, prevents kidney diseases, applies to pets, and boosts exercise performance. Second, highlight the chemistry of sodium bicarbonate, including its composition, reactions, and applications in baking, cleaning, and medicine. Third, highlight the several healing actions and properties due to its alkaline properties and ability to neutralize acids. Fourth, to highlight the devices used to administer sodium bicarbonate to various health conditions. Fifth, to highlight ways baking soda can be consumed in various ways, depending on the intended use. Sixth, highlight several precautions to be taken when using baking soda to treat different health challenges to ensure its safe and effective use. Seventh, highlight the applications in managing and alleviating different health conditions, both in humans and pets.

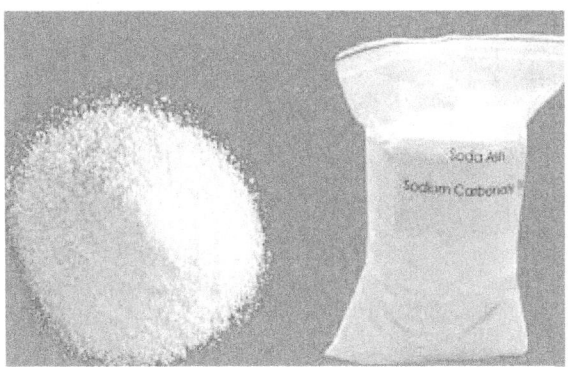

What is baking soda?
Baking soda is a bicarbonate ion "HCO3-" that combines with a sodium cation "Na+". It is used in oral care products for its teeth-whitening and breath-freshening properties. It's also utilized in skincare as a gentle exfoliant and in hair care for various purposes. It's also used in medical treatments under medical supervision. It is a common antacid for heartburn and indigestion since it neutralizes stomach acid. Its use may improve your workout by taking it before you exercise to improve athletic performance in several sports. It shifts inflammatory immune cells in the body to those that combat inflammation when ingested.

Health challenges where healing with baking soda is effective

First, baking soda paste can be applied to minor skin irritations, rashes, and insect bites to relieve itching and inflammation. Second, adding baking soda to a cool bath can provide relief for sunburned skin by soothing and calming the affected area. Third, athletes sometimes use baking soda to reduce exercise-induced acidosis during intense physical activities. It may help improve exercise performance and delay fatigue. Fourth, it may be used under medical supervision to manage specific kidney conditions by reducing acidity in the urine. Fifth, when used with proper medical guidance, it alleviates side effects of chemotherapy, such as oral mucositis, which is inflammation and sores in the mouth. It's essential to use baking soda for health purposes under the guidance of a healthcare professional.

Pros and cons of healing with baking soda

Here are some pros: First, it serves as an antacid to neutralize stomach acid, alleviating the symptoms of heartburn and indigestion. Second, it is a rapid and cost-effective cure for moderate digestive ailments. Third, it helps to relieve itching and pain caused by skin irritations, insect bites, and mild rashes. Fourth, it is used in oral care because of its teeth-whitening and plaque-removing properties, which aid in oral hygiene. Fifth, it is widely available, affordable, and accessible in most households by offering a cost-effective option for health-related remedies. Sixth, it could improve exercise efficiency and prevent fatigue during intense physical activities. Here are some cons: First, excessive use can cause side effects such as gas, bloating, diarrhea, and stomach cramps. Second, excessive use can also upset the body's acid-base balance, resulting in alkalosis, which can have health consequences. Third, it is not utilized in place of professional medical therapy for major medical disorders such as cancer, renal disease, or other chronic illnesses. Fourth, it can interact with certain medications, potentially affecting their absorption or efficacy.

Myths surrounding the uses of baking soda

Some of these myths include: First, several individuals believe baking soda can cure cancer. This is false because this claim can't be proven. Second, individuals believe baking soda can provide a long-term solution for chronic heartburn. In contrast, it can provide temporary relief for heartburn; taking it excessively or too frequently can result in health issues such as electrolyte imbalance and metabolic alkalosis. Third, some individuals believe baking soda whitens teeth instantly. While it is an ingredient in some toothpaste and may assist in removing surface stains, it does not instantly whiten teeth, and its overuse can erode tooth enamel. Fourth, some individuals believe that consuming baking soda can aid in detoxification. However, this is false because its extreme or prolonged consumption can lead to electrolyte imbalances and other health issues. Fifth, some claim that baking soda can replace shampoo for hair cleansing. However, this is not true because using it regularly can disrupt the scalp's pH balance and lead to dryness and damage.

Benefits of using baking soda
Baking soda has several practical and health-related benefits. First, it has household benefits: it is an effective and non-toxic cleaning agent for various surfaces, including countertops, sink, and appliances. It's used to clean and polish silverware, jewelry, and glass surfaces. It can help smother small grease fires. Second, it can be used for personal care benefits; it is used in toothpaste and mouthwash to help whiten teeth and neutralize bad breath. It can relieve skin irritation, insect bites, and sunburn when used in baths or as a paste. It can alleviate foot odor and soften the skin. It may support kidney function by reducing the formation of kidney stones. Third, some athletes use baking soda to help buffer lactic acid and improve exercise endurance. In conclusion, it is essential to consult with a healthcare professional for specific health-related applications and follow recommended guidelines.

CHAPTER TWO

HISTORY OF SODIUM BICARBONATE

Here's a sequential overview of the events in the history of baking soda:

Ancient use of alkaline substances era

Natron, a naturally occurring mixture of sodium carbonate and other salts, was a significant alkaline substance in ancient Egypt. It was harvested from dry lake beds and was a versatile material used in mummification processes, cleaning, and even baking. It was used in cooking and baking, helped dough rise, and contributed to texture and taste. They were used in breaking down oils, fats, and other organic materials, making them valuable for cleaning clothes, tools, and living spaces. They were used in various forms for personal hygiene and cosmetics. Ancient people used mixtures containing alkaline elements for cleansing and beautification purposes. Natron was a vital element in the embalming of bodies during the mummification process in ancient Egypt. Its alkaline properties helped dry out and preserve the remains. They were used to purify water when added to it to neutralize acidity and make the water safer for consumption. They were used in textiles to improve their quality and texture.

The scientific understanding era

In the 18th century, chemists analyzed and experimented with alkaline substances like soda ash and potash. Nicolas Leblanc, a French chemist, invented a process to produce soda ash from common salt. In the early 19th century, Claude-Louis Berthollet, another French chemist, furthered the understanding, including sodium carbonate and potassium carbonate and their applications. Berthollet's research laid the foundation for recognizing the properties and uses of these alkaline compounds.

Leavening in the baking era

The era of leavening in baking with baking soda represented a pivotal period in the history of culinary arts and baking techniques. Leavening agents help dough or batter rise by producing gases (usually carbon dioxide) that get trapped in the mixture, causing it to expand and become lighter. The objective is to have a pleasing texture in the finished baked product.

The commercial production era

In 1946, John Dwight and Austin Church established the first factory to produce baking soda in the United States. This era marked advancements in industrial processes, innovation in production techniques, and the establishment of companies dedicated to the mass production and distribution of baking soda using the Solvay process. Industrialization brought about innovations in the manufacturing process, ensuring higher purity and quality of baking soda by investing in refining techniques, packaging, and distribution to meet evolving consumer demands.

The medicinal use

It worked by neutralizing the acidic environment in the digestive tract as an antacid in the 19th and early 20th centuries. It has been used to help treat certain kidney disorders. It assists in reducing the acidity of urine and may be recommended to help manage conditions that affect kidney function. It has been used for oral health purposes. It is used to help remove plaque and stains from teeth in toothpaste and mouthwash products. It alleviates minor skin irritations, insect bites, and stings. It helped to reduce itching, redness, and discomfort. It helped buffer the boost of lactic acid during intense exercise, delaying fatigue. Research revealed it has an alkalinizing agent to help balance the body's pH levels. It is believed to have potential in cancer treatment as part of an adjunctive therapy.

The widespread usage era
It was used to treat soldiers exposed to chemical warfare during the World War II. Its effectiveness in neutralizing acids makes it valuable for treating burns and exposure to chemical agents. Its role expanded beyond leavening and found applications in tenderizing meat, enhancing the color of vegetables, and

improving the texture of various culinary creations. It was diversified into household cleaning, deodorizing, and personal care. It became a common ingredient in many household products.

The diverse applications era
It became a versatile household staple after the World War. It evolved beyond being solely a leavening agent for baking. Its culinary applications expanded to include tenderizing meat, enhancing the color of vegetables, reducing cooking odors, and serving as a key ingredient in recipes for its unique properties. It was used to clean surfaces, scrub and clean pans, eliminate odors in refrigerators, carpets, shoes, and even unclog drains. It was used to alkalize urine for specific medical conditions and was explored in experimental treatments. It was used to clean and whiten teeth, neutralize mouth odors, and promote healthy gums.

In contemporary times
In contemporary times, it is widely used across various domains due to its versatility, safety, and effectiveness. Its

applications range from culinary uses to cleaning, personal care, health, and more. It is a vital leavening agent in baking. It is used to deodorize fruits and vegetables. It is used as an abrasive cleaner for surfaces like countertops, sinks, and appliances. It is an ingredient in toothpaste and mouthwash due to its teeth-whitening and breath-freshening properties. It is used in natural deodorants to neutralize odor. It's utilized in facial scrubs to exfoliate the skin. It can soothe skin irritation from insect bites and rashes. It's sometimes used in oral rinses to promote a healthy mouth. It is a common ingredient in various scientific experiments and educational demonstrations, showcasing chemical reactions and properties. The contemporary use of baking soda exemplifies its adaptability and a broad spectrum of applications, making it an essential item in households, industries, and personal care regimens.

CHAPTER THREE

THE CHEMISTRY OF SODIUM BICARBONATE

The understanding of the chemical composition and reactions helps explain how baking soda interacts with other substances and its role in baking, cleaning, and medicinal uses.

Chemical structure

It is a white crystalline solid that consists of one sodium ion "Na^+", one bicarbonate ion "HCO_3^-", and one hydrogen ion "H^+". The chemical formula is $NaHCO_3$.

Bicarbonate ion

The bicarbonate ion "HCO_3^-" is a central component of baking soda. It contains one carbon atom "C", one hydrogen atom "H", and three oxygen atoms "O". It acts as a weak base due to its ability to accept a proton "H^+" from an acidic substance.

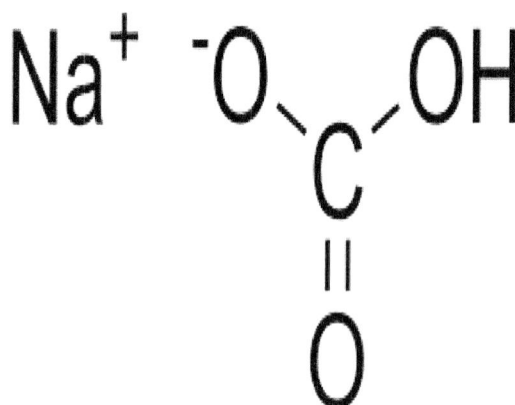

Acid-base properties

In an acidic environment, it behaves as a base by accepting a proton "H+", and in a basic environment, it acts as an acid by donating a proton. Here are equations that demonstrate their amphoteric properties:

As a base in the presence of an acid:

NaHCO3 + HCl → NaCl + H2O + CO2

In this reaction, baking soda "NaHCO3" acts as a base, accepting a proton "H⁺" from hydrochloric acid "HCl" to form sodium chloride "NaCl", water "H2O", and carbon dioxide "CO2".

NaHCO3 + NaOH → Na2CO3 + H2O

In this reaction, baking soda "NaHCO3" acts as an acid, donating a proton "H$^+$" to sodium hydroxide "NaOH" to form sodium carbonate "Na2CO3" and water "H2O".

Reaction with acids

When baking soda reacts with an acid, such as vinegar "acetic acid" or lemon juice "citric acid", it undergoes a chemical reaction. The bicarbonate ion in baking soda reacts with the acid to produce water, carbon dioxide, and a corresponding salt.

Example reaction:

NaHCO3 (s) + CH3COOH (aq) → CO2 (g) + H2O (l) + CH3COONa (aq)

Leavening action in baking

In baking, the reaction of baking soda with an acidic ingredient "such as buttermilk, yogurt" produces carbon dioxide gas. The production of carbon dioxide gas is what creates bubbles and causes the dough or batter to rise, resulting in lighter and fluffier baked goods with the formation of Na$^+$ "Sodium ion", H2O "Water", and CO2.

Here's the equation to illustrate this reaction:

$NaHCO_3 + Acid \rightarrow Na^+ + H_2O + CO_2$

Decomposition at high temperatures

At high temperatures above 50°C or 122°F, baking soda undergoes thermal decomposition, breaking down into sodium carbonate "Na2CO3", water vapor "H2O", and carbon dioxide "CO2". Here's the equation to illustrate this reaction:

$2\ NaHCO_3\ (s) \rightarrow Na_2CO_3\ (s) + H_2O\ (g) + CO_2\ (g)$

Alkalinity and pH regulation

Baking soda can be used to adjust the pH in various applications. When added to an acidic solution, it raises the pH, making it more alkaline. For example, it reacts with HCl "Hydrochloric Acid", which is a component of stomach acid resulting in the formation of NaCl "Sodium Chloride", H2O "Water", and CO2 "Carbon Dioxide Gas". This property is utilized in antacid products to neutralize excess stomach acid, relieving symptoms of heartburn and indigestion. Here's the equation to illustrate this reaction:

$NaHCO_3 + HCl \rightarrow NaCl + H_2O + CO_2$

Sources

Sodium bicarbonate can be sourced from various natural and commercial sources. Here are the primary sources of sodium bicarbonate:

Natural deposits

Sodium bicarbonate occurs naturally in some mineral deposits, such as trona and nahcolite. Trona is primarily found in the Green River Formation in the United States, while nahcolite is mined in areas like the Piceance Basin in Colorado.

Synthetic production

The majority of sodium bicarbonate used commercially is produced synthetically through a chemical reaction between sodium carbonate "soda ash" and carbon dioxide:

$Na_2CO_3 + CO_2 + H_2O \rightarrow 2\ NaHCO_3$

Chemical industries

Chemical manufacturers produce sodium bicarbonate in large quantities through the Solvay process. This process involves reacting sodium chloride "common salt" with ammonia and carbon dioxide. Two molecules of NH3 "Ammonia" and two molecules CO2 "Carbon Dioxide" are reactants that are passed into a solution. NaCl "Sodium Chloride" is also added to the solution resulting in the formation of 2 NH4Cl "Ammonium Chloride" and NaHCO3 "Sodium Bicarbonate". Here's the equation to illustrate this process:

2 NH3 + 2 CO2 + NaCl + 2 H2O → 2 NH4Cl + NaHCO3

Mining and extraction

The extraction of sodium bicarbonate from natural mineral deposits or ore through mining and processing involves several steps. These processes are carried out industrially, and the resulting sodium bicarbonate is then refined and purified for various applications. Here is an equation to illustrate the general concept:

Raw Mineral Deposit → Sodium Bicarbonate

Commercial suppliers
Sodium bicarbonate is widely available from commercial suppliers, both online and in physical stores, in various forms such as powder, granules, tablets, and capsules. These suppliers source the compound from manufacturers and make it available to consumers.

Retail stores
Grocery stores, supermarkets, and stores specializing in baking and cooking ingredients carry sodium bicarbonate as a common household item for baking and other culinary uses.

Extraction Methods
Sodium bicarbonate can be extracted through various methods from natural mineral deposits or through synthetic processes. Here are some extraction methods:

Mining from natural deposits
Sodium bicarbonate can be extracted from natural mineral deposits, such as

trona and nahcolite through mining operations.

Solution mining

Solution mining is a process used to extract sodium bicarbonate from mineral deposits like trona or nahcolite. Here are the simplified chemical equations to illustrate the steps involved in this process:

- First, dissolution in water where sodium bicarbonate "NaHCO3" in the mineral deposit dissolves in water "H2O" in the well as illustrated below

  NaHCO3 (s) + H2O (l) → Na+ (aq) + HCO3- (aq)

- Second, formation of saturated solution where when more water is injected, the solution becomes saturated with sodium bicarbonate, which means no more sodium bicarbonate can dissolve.

$Na^+ (aq) + HCO_3^- (aq) \rightleftharpoons$
$NaHCO_3 (s)$

- Third, bringing the solution to the surface, where the saturated solution is pumped to the surface.
- Fourth, the isolation of sodium bicarbonate through processes such as crystallization and drying.

Solvay process

The Solvay process is a synthetic method for producing sodium bicarbonate from sodium chloride, ammonia, and carbon dioxide. It involves several chemical reactions to ultimately produce sodium bicarbonate:

Reaction with carbon dioxide

Sodium carbonate "soda ash" can react with carbon dioxide and water to produce sodium bicarbonate:

$Na_2CO_3 + CO_2 + H_2O \rightarrow 2\ NaHCO_3$

Neutralization reaction

Sodium bicarbonate can be produced through a neutralization reaction between sodium hydroxide "caustic soda" and carbon dioxide:

NaOH + CO2 → NaHCO3

Electrolysis

The production of baking soda by electrolysis involves passing an electric current through a concentrated sodium chloride solution to separate sodium ions and bicarbonate ions. The process at the cathode reduces water "H_2O" to produce hydrogen gas "H_2" and hydroxide ions "OH^-", while at the anode, chloride ions "Cl^-" are oxidized to form chlorine gas "Cl_2" and release electrons "$2e^-$". These reactions result in the generation of hydroxide ions, which then combine with sodium ions to form sodium hydroxide "NaOH". This sodium hydroxide can be used to react with carbon dioxide to produce baking soda. Here are the chemical equations:

Cathode (Reduction):

$$2H_2O(l) + 2e^- \rightarrow H_2(g) + 2OH^-(aq)$$

Anode (Oxidation):

$$2Cl^-(aq) \rightarrow Cl_2(g) + 2e^-$$

Overall Reactions:

$2H_2O(l) + 2Cl^-(aq) \rightarrow H_2(g) + Cl_2(g) + 2OH^-(aq)$

2 NaCl (aq) + 2 H2O (l) + 2 e⁻ → 2 NaOH (aq) + Cl2 (g) + H2 (g)

NaOH + CO2 → NaHCO3

Where,

2 NaCl (aq) represents sodium chloride dissolved in water.

2 H2O (l) is water.

2 e⁻ represents the electrons that are supplied through the electrical current.

2 NaOH (aq) is sodium hydroxide, which is formed during the electrolysis.

Cl2 (g) is chlorine gas, which is one of the products of the electrolysis.

H2 (g) is hydrogen gas, another product of the electrolysis.

Purification and crystallization

Once the sodium bicarbonate is obtained through the above methods, it undergoes purification and crystallization processes to isolate the compound in its desired form, such as powder or granules.

Grades

Sodium bicarbonate is available in various grades based on its purity, intended use, and compliance with specific industry or regulatory standards. Here are the common grades of sodium bicarbonate:

Food grade

Food grade sodium bicarbonate is the highest quality and purity suitable for consumption. It meets the strict standards set by food regulatory bodies and is commonly used in cooking, baking, and other food-related applications.

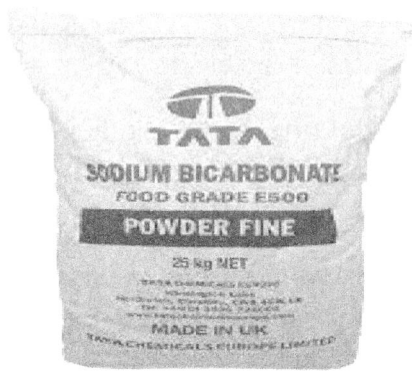

Pharmaceutical grade

Pharmaceutical grade sodium bicarbonate is of high purity and meets the standards specified for medicinal and pharmaceutical purposes. It is used in antacid formulations and certain medical treatments under the supervision of healthcare professionals.

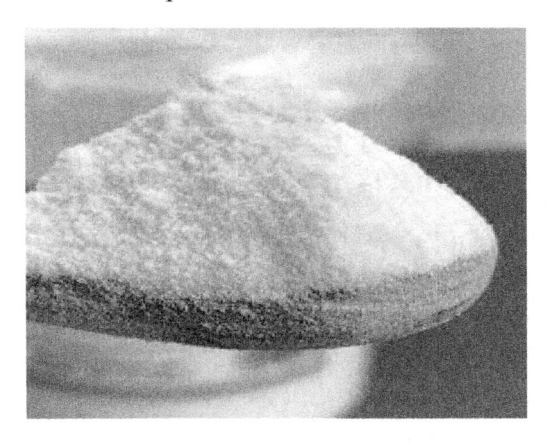

United States Pharmacopeia grade

Sodium bicarbonate that complies with the standards set by the United States Pharmacopeia (USP) for quality and purity. It is suitable for use in pharmaceutical and medicinal products.

Technical grade

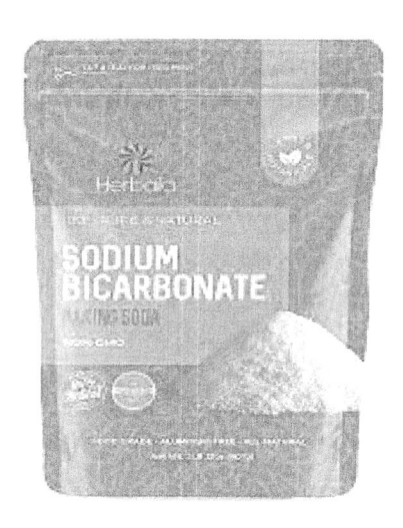

Technical grade sodium bicarbonate is of a lower purity compared to food and pharmaceutical grades. It is intended for industrial and technical applications such as water treatment, fire extinguishing systems, cleaning agents, and other industrial processes.

Industrial grade

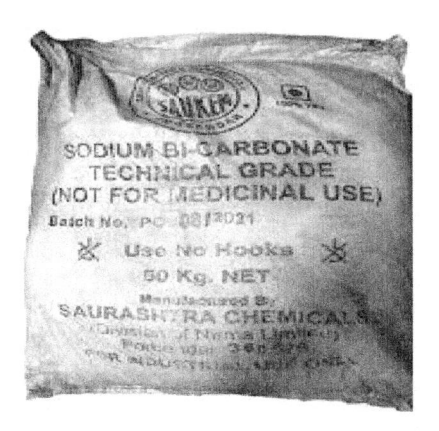

Industrial grade sodium bicarbonate is generally used in a variety of industrial applications. It may have a lower purity compared to other grades and is suitable for uses such as water treatment, flue gas desulfurization, detergent production, and more.

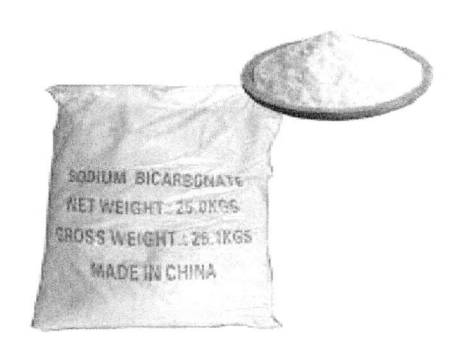

Agricultural grade
Sodium bicarbonate in this grade is used in agricultural applications, including soil amendments and animal feed supplements. It helps control pH levels in the soil and promotes healthy plant growth.

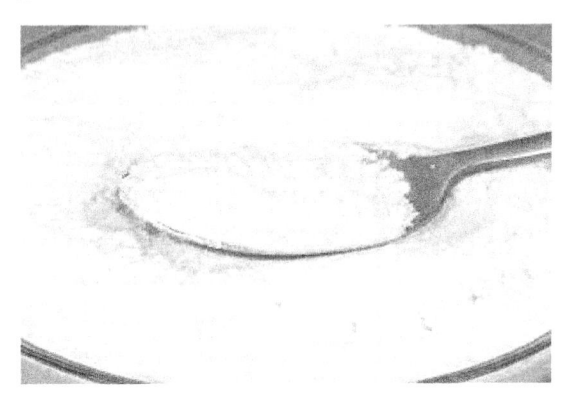

Reagent grade
Reagent grade sodium bicarbonate is of high purity and is used in laboratory settings, chemical analysis, and scientific research where precise measurements and purity are significant.

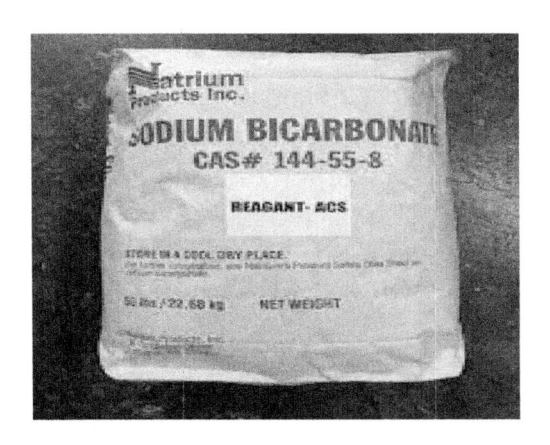

Cosmetic grade

This grade meets specific purity and safety standards for cosmetic and personal care product applications. It is used in products such as toothpaste, mouthwash, deodorants, and skin care formulations.

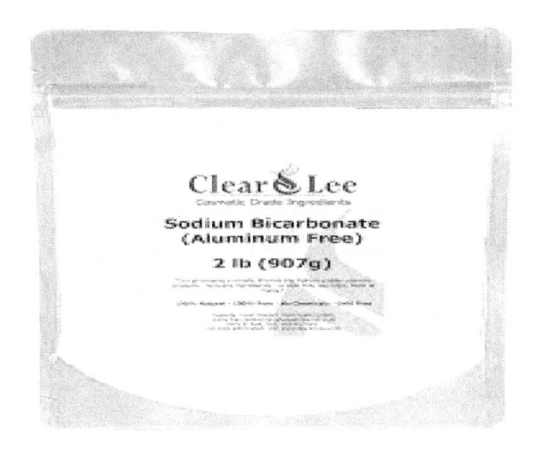

Specialty grades
Specialty grades of sodium bicarbonate may be tailored to specific applications or industries, incorporating additional properties or characteristics to meet specialized needs.

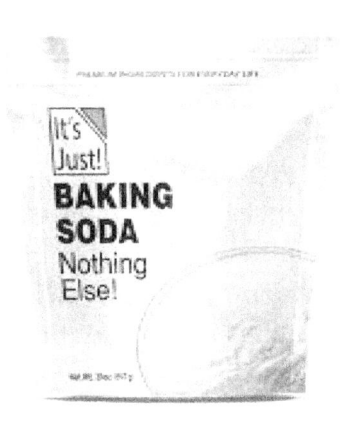

Properties
Here are the properties of sodium bicarbonate:

Physical properties
It possesses several distinctive physical properties. These properties contribute to its versatility and functionality in various applications. Here are the physical properties of baking soda:

- It is a fine, white, crystalline powder.
- It appears as a white, opaque substance in its powdered form.
- The powder is soft with a powdery texture, making it dispersible and mixable.
- It has a slightly alkaline taste and a mild, salty flavor.
- It is odorless when dry.
- It is soluble in water.
- It undergoes decomposition before melting. At an approximate temperature of 50°C "122°F",
- It begins to decompose into sodium carbonate, water, and carbon dioxide.
- The density of baking soda ranges from about 2.20 to 2.50 grams per cubic centimeter "g/cm^3"
- It is slightly alkaline, with a pH of around 8.3 in a 1% aqueous solution.
- The particle size of baking soda powder varies, but it is generally very fine, allowing for even distribution in various applications.

- Its crystals belong to the monoclinic crystal system, characterized by three unequal crystallographic axes.

Chemical properties

Here are the chemical properties of baking soda:

- It can react with acids, forming water and salt, or with bases to yield water and a carbonate ion.
- It reacts with acids to produce carbon dioxide, water, and salt. For instance: $NaHCO_3 + HCl \rightarrow CO_2 + H_2O + NaCl$
- It undergoes thermal decomposition at temperatures above 50°C "122°F", breaking down into sodium carbonate "Na_2CO_3", water "H_2O", and carbon dioxide "CO_2". $2NaHCO_3 \rightarrow Na_2CO_3 + H_2O + CO_2$
- It can neutralize acids, helping to balance pH levels. Adding to an acidic solution raises the pH, acting as an antacid.

- It reacts with an acid to produce carbon dioxide gas, leading to effervescence. This property is essential for its leavening action in baking.
- It can undergo carbonation when exposed to carbon dioxide, forming sodium carbonate and water: $NaHCO_3 + CO_2 \rightarrow Na_2CO_3 + H_2O$
- It exhibits buffering properties, helping to stabilize the pH of a solution by resisting changes in acidity or alkalinity.
- It dissolves in water, and when dissolved, it dissociates into sodium ions "Na^+", bicarbonate ions "HCO_3^-", and hydroxide ions "OH^-".
- It can participate in redox reactions, although it is more involved in acid-base reactions.
- It is stable under normal conditions but can undergo degradation if exposed to heat, moisture, or acidic environments for extended periods.

Laboratory preparation

Here's a commonly used method for laboratory preparation:

Using sodium carbonate and carbon dioxide

Materials and chemicals:

- Sodium carbonate "Na2CO3"
- Carbon dioxide "CO2" source by reacting an acid with a carbonate

Procedure:

- First, mix the sodium carbonate with water to create slurry. Ensure thorough mixing to dissolve the sodium carbonate as much as possible.
- Second, pass carbon dioxide gas through the slurry. This can be done by bubbling CO2 through the slurry using a delivery tube.
- Third, continue bubbling CO2 until no more gas is absorbed, and a white precipitate of sodium bicarbonate forms in the solution.

- Fourth, filter the solution to separate the precipitated sodium bicarbonate from the liquid.
- Fifth, rinse the precipitate with cold water to remove impurities.
- Sixth, dry the obtained sodium bicarbonate in an oven.
  $Na_2CO_3 + CO_2 + H_2O \rightarrow 2 NaHCO_3$
  In this reaction, sodium carbonate reacts with carbon dioxide and water to produce sodium bicarbonate.

The commercial production

The commercial production involves the Solvay process, which is a well-established and highly efficient industrial method. Here's a detailed outline of it:

Raw materials
- Sodium chloride "common salt"
- Ammonia "NH3"
- Carbon dioxide "CO2"
- Water "H2O"

First step: formation of sodium bicarbonate

The first step in the Solvay process involves the formation of sodium hydrogen carbonate from sodium chloride, ammonia, and carbon dioxide.

Ammonia reacts with common salt:

In this reaction, ammonia "NH3" reacts with sodium chloride "NaCl" to produce ammonium chloride "NH4Cl".

NH3 (aq) + NaCl (aq) → NH4Cl (aq)

Carbon dioxide is introduced:

In this equation below, ammonium chloride "NH4Cl" reacts with sodium carbonate "Na2CO3" in the presence of water and carbon dioxide "CO2". The result is the formation of sodium bicarbonate "NaHCO3" and the regeneration of ammonium chloride "NH4Cl".

NH4Cl (aq) + Na2CO3 (s) + H2O (l) + 2 CO2 (g) → 2 NaHCO3 (aq) + 2 NH4Cl (aq)

Second step: regeneration of ammonium chloride

The ammonium chloride formed in the first step is recycled back into the process:

Ammonium chloride recovery:

Ammonium chloride is heated with calcium oxide "CaO", releasing ammonia gas "NH3" and forming calcium chloride "CaCl2" and water "H2O". The ammonia gas is reused in the first step.

2 NH4Cl (aq) + CaO (s) → 2 NH3 (g) + CaCl2 (aq) + H2O (l)

Third step: recovery of sodium carbonate

To complete the Solvay process, the sodium carbonate is regenerated for further use:

Recovery of sodium carbonate:

Sodium bicarbonate "NaHCO3" is treated with calcium hydroxide "Ca (OH) 2" to regenerate sodium carbonate "Na2CO3", water "H2O", and calcium carbonate "CaCO3". The sodium carbonate can be used as the final product or processed further for specific applications, including the production of baking soda.

2 NaHCO3 (aq) + Ca (OH) 2 (aq) → 2 Na2CO3 (aq) + 2 H2O (l) + CaCO3 (s)

CHAPTER FOUR

HEALING ACTIONS AND PROPERTIES

Baking soda has several healing actions due to its alkaline properties and ability to neutralize acids.

Antacid properties

The antacid properties of baking soda lie in its ability to neutralize excess stomach acid. When consumed, it reacts with the hydrochloric acid in the stomach to form salt, water, and carbon dioxide gas. The sodium bicarbonate "NaHCO3" reacts with hydrochloric acid "HCl" in the stomach, forming sodium chloride "NaCl" water "H2O", and carbon dioxide gas "CO2". The release of carbon dioxide can cause gas, providing temporary relief from symptoms of heartburn, indigestion, and acid reflux.

NaHCO3 + HCl → NaCl + H2O + CO2

Abrasive properties

Its mild abrasive properties help remove plaque and stains from teeth, and its alkaline nature can also help neutralize acids in the mouth when used in toothpaste and mouthwash to promote oral hygiene and white teeth. It is sometimes included in skin care routines as an ingredient in exfoliating scrubs. Its gentle abrasiveness helps kill skin cells, leaving the skin feeling refreshed.

Anti-inflammatory and soothing properties

Its anti-inflammatory and soothing properties may help relieve skin irritations, itching, and minor rashes when applied topically in a paste or added to bath water to soothe skin. Its mild abrasive properties and its fine, powdery texture in the context of personal care are often utilized in toothpaste and mouthwash to help remove surface stains from teeth. It aids in polishing and scrubbing away plaque and stains without causing significant damage to the tooth enamel. It is sometimes included in skin care routines as an ingredient in exfoliating scrubs. Its gentle abrasiveness helps remove dead skin cells, leaving the skin smooth and refreshed.

Antifungal and odor-neutralizing properties

Its antifungal and odor-neutralizing properties can help with foot hygiene and minimize foot odor when added to foot soaks or used in powder form in shoes. It helps by absorbing moisture, thus reducing the environment where odor-causing bacteria can thrive. It also neutralizes the acidic compounds responsible for the unpleasant smell.

Alkaline properties

Its alkaline properties may help alleviate itching and irritation from insect bites and stings when baking soda and water are applied to the affected area. When dissolved in water, it forms a solution that can neutralize acids, raising the pH level. It reacts with acids to form water, salt, and carbon dioxide gas. This reaction helps neutralize acids and reduce their impact. It's used as an antacid for conditions like heartburn and acid reflux. When added to a solution, it raises the pH, making it more alkaline. This property is utilized in cleaning, skincare, and other applications that benefit from a more alkaline environment. Its alkalinity contributes to its ability to absorb and neutralize acidic odors, as it interacts with and neutralizes acidic compounds that cause unpleasant smells.

Alkalization properties

The alkalizing properties of baking soda refer to its ability to increase the pH of a substance, making it more alkaline or basic. This is due to the nature of baking soda, a weak alkaline compound that can elevate the pH level when introduced into a solution. Its alkalization properties help to alkalinize the urine, which is beneficial for people with certain urinary tract conditions when used under medical supervision for specific urinary issues. Some people use it to help alkalize the body, believing that maintaining an alkaline pH may offer health benefits. However, altering the body's pH should be done cautiously and under professional guidance. In the digestive system, it acts as an antacid, neutralizing excess stomach acid, raising the pH level in the stomach, and providing relief from heartburn and indigestion. Its alkalization properties are utilized to soothe minor skin irritations and sunburn when used in baths or as a paste. It can help balance the skin's pH, providing relief.

Buffering capacity

Athletes sometimes use baking soda as an ergogenic aid to enhance exercise performance and delay fatigue. The theory behind this usage lies in the compound's buffering capacity. Lactic acid is produced as an aftermath of anaerobic metabolism during vigorous exercise. Lactic acid buildup can lead to muscle fatigue and a decrease in performance. As a base, it can act as a buffer, neutralizing excess lactic acid that accumulates in the muscles during strenuous activity. It helps delay the onset of muscle fatigue and the associated discomfort, allowing athletes to sustain intense effort for a longer duration before experiencing exhaustion.

CHAPTER FIVE

DEVICES FOR USE WITH SODIUM BICARBONATE

Sodium bicarbonate can be used in with various devices for administering it to different health conditions.

Devices and methods

Here are some devices used with sodium bicarbonate:

Nebulizers

Administering sodium bicarbonate through a nebulizer for individuals to manage respiratory acidosis requires a specialized medical procedure that should only be conducted under the supervision and guidance of a healthcare professional. Here are some general steps one might follow:

- First, assemble the nebulizer according to the manufacturer's instructions. Ensure the nebulizer

is clean, sterilized, and in proper working condition.
- Second, measure the sodium bicarbonate solution dose prescribed by your healthcare provider.
- Third, if the sodium bicarbonate solution requires dilution, follow the instructions given by your healthcare provider or pharmacist.
- Fourth, pour the sodium bicarbonate solution into the nebulizer's medication cup.
- Fifth, attach the appropriate mask to the nebulizer based on the patient's age and medical recommendations.
- Sixth, for optimal lung function, sit upright on it, turn on the nebulizer, and inhale the sodium bicarbonate mist as directed by your healthcare provider. Breathe calmly and deeply through the mouth until all the medication is administered.
- Finally, continue using the nebulizer until the prescribed sodium bicarbonate dose is

delivered according to your healthcare provider's instructions.

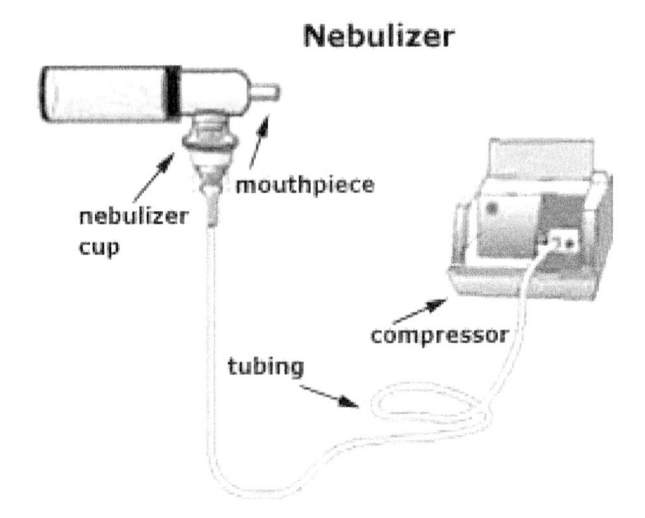

Nebulizer

Intravenous administration devices

Here are the steps that healthcare professionals would follow when using intravenous administration devices to administer sodium bicarbonate:

- First, assemble all the necessary supplies, including a vial or pre-filled syringe of sodium bicarbonate, intravenous tubing,

a compatible infusion pump, alcohol swabs, and gloves.
- Second, review the physician's order and confirm the correct dosage and concentration of sodium bicarbonate to be administered.
- Third, perform proper hand hygiene and wear appropriate personal protective equipment (PPE), such as gloves.
- Fourth, if using a vial, withdraw the required dose of sodium bicarbonate using a sterile syringe. If using a pre-filled syringe, verify the dosage and concentration.
- Fifth, confirm the compatibility of the sodium bicarbonate with the intravenous solution, if applicable. Double-check the dose against the prescription.
- Sixth, attach the sodium bicarbonate-filled syringe or vial to the appropriate injection port on the intravenous line or extension tubing.

- Seventh, prime the intravenous line to remove air bubbles and ensure medication flows smoothly.
- Eighth, administer the sodium bicarbonate at the prescribed rate using an infusion pump, according to the healthcare provider's instructions.
- Ninth, continuously monitor the patient's vital signs, infusion rate, and response to the medication.
- Tenth, administer the entire prescribed dose of sodium bicarbonate and document the administration, including the time, patient's response, and adverse reactions.
- Eleventh, safely dispose of any used equipment and waste following appropriate medical waste disposal protocols.
- Finally, monitor the patient for any adverse reactions or complications associated with the administration.

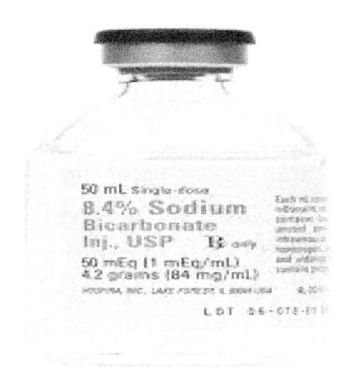

Gastrointestinal tubes

Here are the steps that healthcare professionals would follow when using gastrointestinal tubes to administer sodium bicarbonate:

- First, assess the patient's medical condition, vital signs, and suitability for gastrointestinal tube administration of sodium bicarbonate based on the physician's order.
- Second, review the physician's order for the prescribed dosage and prepare the appropriate dose according to the order.

- Third, confirm the compatibility of the sodium bicarbonate with the gastrointestinal tube and any other medications the patient may be receiving. Dilute the sodium bicarbonate as needed based on the order.
- Fourth, confirm the correct placement and positioning of the gastrointestinal tube using appropriate techniques, such as X-rays or pH testing.
- Fifth, flush the gastrointestinal tube with a small amount of water or saline solution to ensure it is clear and functional.
- Sixth, attach a syringe filled with the prepared sodium bicarbonate solution to the appropriate port on the gastrointestinal tube.
- Seventh, administer the sodium bicarbonate solution slowly and gently through the gastrointestinal tube as per the prescribed rate and duration.
- Eighth, flush the gastrointestinal tube again with water or saline solution to ensure the complete

delivery of sodium bicarbonate and prevent blockages.
- Ninth, monitor the patient for any discomfort, adverse reactions, or complications during and after the administration.
- Tenth, document the administration of sodium bicarbonate, including the dose, time, patient's response, and any adverse reactions.
- Finally, educate the patient or caregiver about the procedure, the purpose of sodium bicarbonate administration, potential side effects, and any necessary follow-up care.

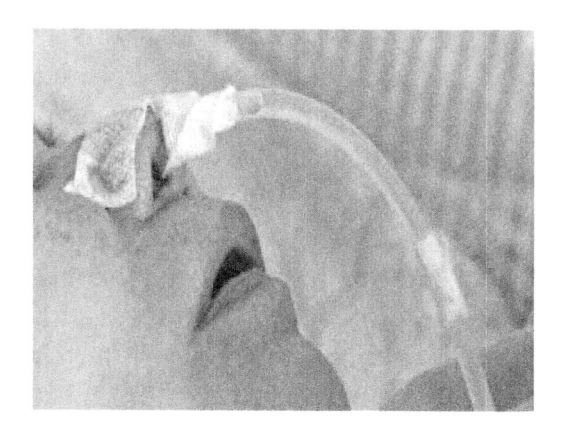

Dental applications

Dental applications such as toothbrushes and mouthwash dispensers play an essential role in oral care and teeth whitening. Here are steps on how to use these tools effectively for oral hygiene and teeth whitening:

Using a toothbrush for oral hygiene

- First, select a toothbrush with soft bristles and an appropriate size for your mouth. Soft bristles help prevent damage to gums and tooth enamel.
- Second, squeeze a pea-sized amount of fluoride toothpaste onto the toothbrush bristles.
- Third, wet the toothbrush under running water to moisten the bristles.
- Fourth, hold the toothbrush at a 45-degree angle to your gum line. Brush the exterior and inner surfaces of your teeth with gentle, circular strokes. For the chewing surfaces, use a back-and-forth motion. Brush your tongue and

the roof of your mouth to reduce bacteria.
- Fifth, brush your teeth for at least two minutes to ensure a thorough cleaning.
- Sixth, after brushing, rinse your mouth with water or mouthwash to remove any residual toothpaste.
- Seventh, replace your toothbrush every three months or sooner if the bristles appear worn.

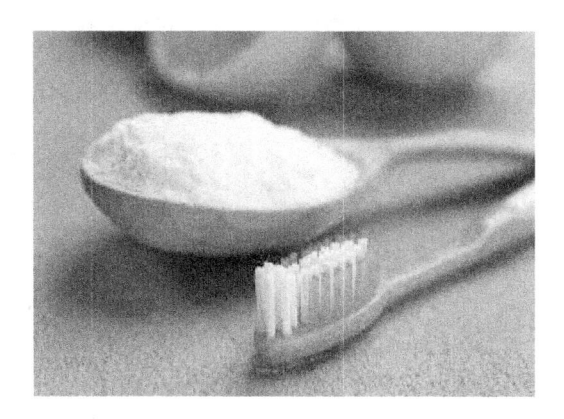

Using a mouthwash dispenser

- First, select a mouthwash that suits your needs, whether for fresh breath, cavity prevention, or teeth whitening.

- Second, use the marked dispenser to measure the recommended amount of mouthwash.
- Third, pour the measured mouthwash into the dispenser.
- Fourth, pre-rinse with water before using the mouthwash. Follow the instructions on the mouthwash label.
- Fifth, take the mouthwash into your mouth and swish it around for about 45 seconds. Rinse your mouth with the mouthwash for a few seconds in the back of your throat.
- Sixth, spit out the mouthwash into the sink.
- Seventh, avoid eating or drinking for thirty minutes after using a mouthwash to allow the active ingredients to work effectively.
- Seventh, follow the usage instructions on the label, which may vary based on the specific mouthwash.

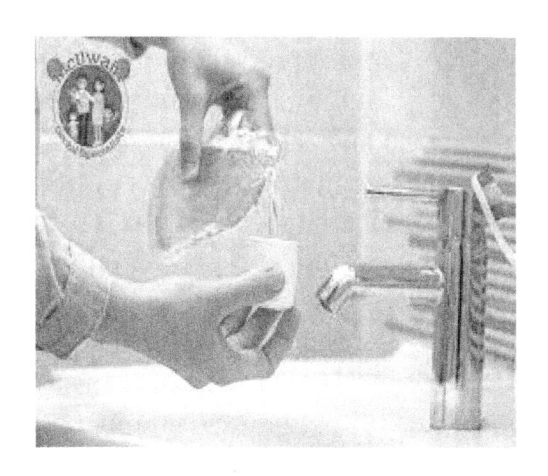

Infusion pumps for urinary alkalinization

Here are the steps that healthcare professionals would follow when using infusion pumps for this purpose:

- First, assess the patient's medical condition, history of drug overdose or poisoning, renal function, electrolyte levels, and acid-base balance.
- Second, review the physician's order for the prescribed rate and concentration of sodium bicarbonate for urinary alkalinization and prepare the

appropriate sodium bicarbonate solution based on the order.
- Third, confirm the compatibility and appropriateness of the sodium bicarbonate solution for urinary alkalinization based on the patient's condition and the drug ingested. Dilute the sodium bicarbonate solution as needed, following the recommended guidelines.
- Fourth, set up the infusion pump and ensure it is calibrated accurately to deliver the prescribed rate of sodium bicarbonate solution.
- Fifth, insert the intravenous line into a suitable vein in the patient's arm or other appropriate site. Start the infusion pump to administer the sodium bicarbonate solution at the prescribed rate.
- Sixth, monitor the infusion to ensure proper flow and infusion rate according to the physician's order.
- Seventh, monitor the urine pH periodically to ensure the desired

alkalinization effect is achieved. Adjust the infusion rate of sodium bicarbonate as needed to maintain the target urine pH.
- Eighth, regularly monitor the patient's electrolyte levels, particularly serum bicarbonate, to evaluate the effectiveness of urinary alkalinization. Adjust the sodium bicarbonate infusion rate or concentration based on monitoring results.
- Ninth, administer the entire amount of sodium bicarbonate per the healthcare provider's instructions. Document the administration, including the dose, rate, duration, urine pH, and patient's response.
- Finally, continuously monitor the patient's response and adjust the infusion rate or other interventions as necessary.

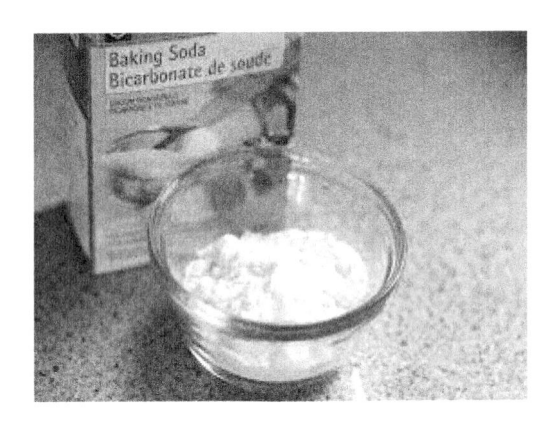

Skin and scalp applicators

Here are the steps on how to use skin and scalp applicators:

- First, start by cleaning the affected area with mild soap and water and dry with a towel.
- Second, examine the skin to identify the affected areas, such as insect bites, minor irritations, or sunburn.
- Third, select an appropriate topical solution or cream to relieve skin irritations, insect bites, or sunburn.
- Fourth, read the instructions and guidelines on the product label to understand the proper application

method and any specific precautions.
- Fifth, dispense a small amount of the topical solution onto the applicator (a cotton ball, swab, or your fingers), depending on the product's instructions.
- Sixth, gently apply the topical solution to the affected areas, covering the entire area with a thin layer. Avoid excessive rubbing or scratching.
- Seventh, massage the solution into the skin or gently dab the affected areas to aid absorption and ensure even distribution.
- Eighth, let the solution be absorbed by the skin by allowing the skin to air-dry for a few minutes.
- Ninth, depending on the product instructions, reapply the topical solution as needed to maintain relief and comfort.
- Tenth, monitor the affected areas for improvement or signs of allergic reactions.

- Finally, encourage the individual to avoid scratching the affected area to prevent further irritation.

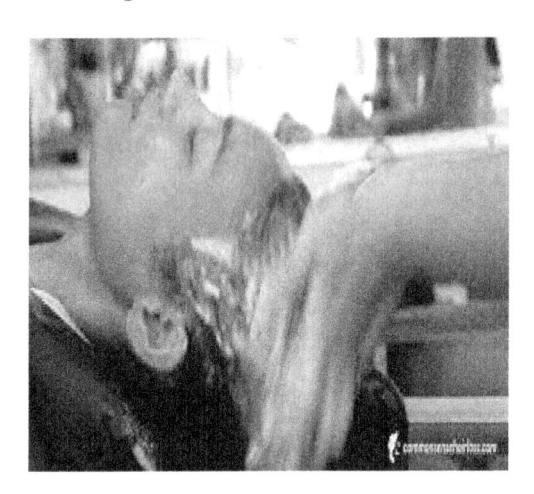

Sprayers for oral conditions

Here are the steps on how to use sprayers for the mouth or throat:

- First, choose a spray product such as sore throat spray or mouth ulcer spray.
- Second, read the product instructions carefully to understand the specific usage guidelines, dosage, and precautions.

- Third, some sprays may require shaking the bottle before use. Check the product instructions for this information.
- Fourth, ensure proper hand hygiene by washing your hands before handling the sprayer or placing anything in your mouth.
- Fifth, open your mouth wide to facilitate easy access to the sprayer.
- Sixth, aim the sprayer nozzle toward the affected area in your mouth or throat.
- Seventh, depress the sprayer button or pump to release the spray.
- Eighth, while aiming the spray, press the sprayer to deliver the recommended dosage.
- Ninth, follow the instructions regarding whether to swallow the spray or gargle with it.
- Tenth, after spraying, close your mouth and avoid swallowing for a short period as directed by the product instructions.

- Eleventh, depending on the product, avoid eating or drinking for a specified time after using the spray to allow it to take effect.
- Twelfth, clean the sprayer according to the product instructions to maintain hygiene and prevent contamination.
- Finally, store the sprayer in a cool, dry, and keep it away from direct sunlight or extreme temperatures.

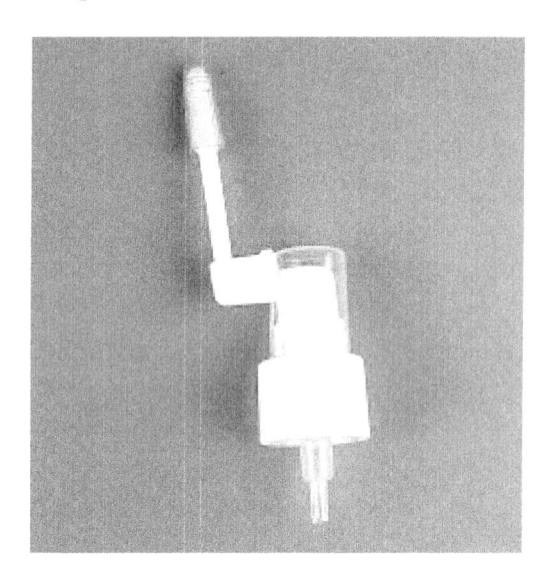

CHAPTER SIX

FORMS BAKING SODA CAN BE CONSUMED

Baking soda can be consumed in various ways depending on the intended use.

Baking soda solution

To prepare and consume a baking soda solution for potential relief from health conditions, follow these steps:

- First, gather supplies: a clean glass, a measuring spoon, and baking soda.
- Second, use a measuring spoon to measure the desired amount of baking soda. The dosage is half to one teaspoon of baking soda.
- Third, prepare a glass by placing the measured baking soda in the clean glass.
- Fourth, fill the glass with about 240 ml of cold water.
- Fifth, stir the mixture well to ensure the baking soda is completely dissolved in the water.

- Sixth, drink the baking soda solution slowly. Do not consume it all at once; sip it over a few minutes.
- Seventh, after consuming the solution, wait for potential relief from symptoms.
- Finally, pay attention to how your body responds to the solution. Note any improvement in symptoms or potential adverse effects.

Baking soda paste

Here are the steps to make and apply a baking soda paste:

- First, gather supplies by getting baking soda and a small bowl or container for mixing.
- Second, measure the desired amount of baking soda based on the intended use. Usually, one or two teaspoons are sufficient.
- Third, slowly add a small amount of water to the baking soda, a few drops at a time, and mix until you achieve a thick, spreadable paste.

- Fourth, use a spoon or fork to thoroughly mix the baking soda and water until a smooth paste is formed.
- Fifth, adjust the amount of water or baking soda to achieve the desired consistency.
- Sixth, using clean fingers, apply the baking soda paste to the affected area. Spread it evenly.
- Seventh, allow the paste to remain on the skin for about 15 minutes.
- Eighth, gently rinse the area with warm water to remove the paste.
- Finally, pat the skin dry with a clean towel.

Cooking and baking

Here are steps to properly use baking soda in cooking and baking:

- First, understand that it is a leavening agent that requires an acid such as yogurt, vinegar, or lemon juice to activate and produce carbon dioxide gas, causing dough or batter to rise.
- Second, choose a recipe that calls for baking soda as an ingredient.

Recipes include cakes, cookies, pancakes, quick breads, and muffins.
- Third, read and follow the recipe instructions carefully, including the specified amount of baking soda needed.
- Fourth, use a dry measuring spoon to measure the precise amount of baking soda specified in the recipe.
- Fifth, combine with dry ingredients such as "flour, salt, etc." before adding wet ingredients. This ensures even distribution.
- Sixth, mix the dry ingredients, including the baking soda, to ensure they are evenly distributed.
- Seventh, put the wet ingredients, such as eggs, milk, and oil, into the dry mixture and mix until combined.
- Eighth, preheat the oven to the specified temperature in the recipe and bake according to the instructions.

- Finally, observe how the dough or batter rises, achieving a light and fluffy texture due to the carbon dioxide released by the baking soda.

Oral rinse

Using baking soda as an oral rinse can help neutralize acids in the mouth and freshen your breath. Here are the steps to follow:

- First, get baking soda and a clean glass for mixing.
- Second, measure half to one teaspoon of baking soda.
- Third, place the measured baking soda in a clean glass.
- Fourth, fill the glass with about 240 ml of warm water.
- Fifth, stir the mixture until the baking soda is dissolved.
- Sixth, take a sip from the solution and gargle for about thirty seconds.
- Seventh, spit out into the sink.

- Eighth, rinse your mouth with water to remove residual baking soda taste.
- Finally, you can repeat the process at least once daily for oral freshness.

Toothpaste

Using baking soda as toothpaste can help with oral hygiene and freshness. Here are steps to create and use baking soda toothpaste:

- First, get baking soda, water, a small bowl, and a clean toothbrush.
- Second, measure a small amount of baking soda, about a pea-sized amount.
- Third, put the measured baking soda in a small bowl.
- Fourth, add a few drops of water to the baking soda to create a paste-like consistency. Start with a minimal amount and gradually add more if needed.
- Fifth, mix the baking soda and water until you achieve a smooth

paste. The goal is to make a spreadable paste.
- Sixth, insert your toothbrush into the baking soda paste, ensuring the bristles are coated.
- Seventh, brush your teeth using the baking soda paste focusing on all surfaces of your teeth, and brush for about two minutes.
- Eighth, spit out the paste and rinse your mouth thoroughly with water to remove any residual baking soda.
- Finally, use this baking soda paste instead of your regular toothpaste, as desired or as recommended by your dentist.

Antacid tablets

Here are the steps to use baking soda as an antacid tablet:

- First, gather supplies by getting baking soda and water.
- Second, measure half a teaspoon to one teaspoon of baking soda.
- Third, put the measured baking soda into a clean glass.

- Fourth, fill the glass with about 240 ml of cold water.
- Fifth, stir the mixture until the baking soda is dissolved in the water.
- Sixth, drink the baking soda solution slowly.

Supplements

Baking soda supplements, in the form of capsules or tablets, are available and can be consumed as directed for medical conditions under the guidance of a healthcare professional. Here are the steps:

- First, consult with a healthcare provider to provide guidance based on your health conditions.
- Second, work with your healthcare professional to determine the appropriate dosage of baking soda as a supplement.
- Third, measure the amount of baking soda recommended.
- Fourth, mix the measured baking soda with water to create a solution for easier consumption.

- Fifth, take the baking soda solution as directed by your healthcare provider.

Beverage additive

To use it as beverage additives add a small amount of baking soda to beverages like water or tea, especially for potential relief from acid reflux and heartburn, to adjust the acidity, or to create a carbonated effect, follow these steps:

- First, gather supplies by getting baking soda and the beverage of your choice.
- Second, measure the desired amount of baking soda.
- Third, choose a beverage such as water, juice, or a smoothie to which you'll add the baking soda.
- Fourth, sprinkle or add the measured baking soda to the beverage.
- Fifth, stir the beverage well to ensure the baking soda is dissolved and evenly distributed.
- Sixth, taste the beverage and adjust the amount of baking soda

if needed to achieve the desired taste.
- Finally, drink the beverage with the baking soda added.

Dissolved in juice

To dissolve in juice, mix a small amount of baking soda to help cover the taste and consume it for potential relief from gastrointestinal discomfort. Here are the steps to follow:

- First, gather supplies by getting baking soda and the juice of your choice.
- Second, measure the desired amount of baking soda.
- Fourth, sprinkle the measured baking soda into the juice.
- Fifth, stir the juice well to ensure the baking soda is dissolved and evenly distributed.
- Finally, drink the juice with the baking soda added.

CHAPTER SEVEN

PRECAUTIONS

This chapter highlights several precautions to be taken when using baking soda to treat different health challenges to ensure its safe and effective use.

Consulting healthcare professional

Here are some tips to help you approach a consultation with a healthcare professional regarding the use of sodium bicarbonate:

- First, have a clear understanding of why you are considering its use by researching the uses, benefits, and risks of using baking soda.
- Second, gather information about your medical history, present health condition, any medications or supplements you're taking and any allergies you may have. Also, note down your symptoms.

- Third, depending on your needs, consult an appropriate healthcare professional.
- Fourth, be honest and transparent by being open about your intentions and concerns regarding providing a complete and accurate medical history, including any previous experiences with it.
- Fifth, prepare a list of questions you will ask the healthcare professional, such as potential benefits, risks, dosage, interactions, and alternative treatments.
- Sixth, share the findings of the research you've conducted and discuss your concerns regarding using sodium bicarbonate. Seek the healthcare professional's opinion and advice based on your specific situation.
- Seventh, listen carefully to the healthcare professional's advice and recommendations. Follow their instructions regarding dosage, administration, frequency, and any precautions.

- Eighth, ensure to discuss any underlying medical conditions you have and the medications you're currently taking.
- Ninth, discuss alternative treatment options if sodium bicarbonate is not recommended or suitable for your situation.
- Tenth, ask about follow-up appointment intervals for checking progress or adjusting the treatment plan.
- Eleventh, don't hesitate to ask for further clarification or more information.
- Finally, adhere to the healthcare professional's recommendations and instructions.

Dosage and administration

Here are some tips:

- First, consult a healthcare professional to determine the appropriate dosage and administration of sodium bicarbonate based on your

specific health condition, medical history, and current medications.
- Second, adhere strictly to the dosage and administration guidelines provided by your healthcare professional.
- Third, understand the specific health condition being treated and how sodium bicarbonate may address it.
- Fourth, the dosage may vary based on the concentration. Dosage for oral use and antacid use to relieve heartburn or indigestion: adult dosage is half to one teaspoon "2.5 to 5 grams" dissolved in a glass of water, usually every two to four hours.
- Fifth, administer it according to the directed frequency and duration specified.
- Sixth, avoid exceeding the recommended dosage; it can lead to electrolyte imbalances and other health issues.
- Seventh, your healthcare provider may monitor your progress and adjust the dosage accordingly.

- Eighth, dosages may need adjustment for children or those with certain medical conditions. Follow healthcare advice.
- Ninth, avoid mixing sodium bicarbonate with acidic substances, as this can neutralize its effectiveness.
- Tenth, if using it for oral hygiene, follow dental guidelines and consult a dentist for appropriate dosage and administration.

Avoid prolonged use

Here are some tips to avoid prolonged use:

- First, consult a healthcare professional to determine the appropriate duration.
- Second, strictly follow the recommended duration and dosage guidelines provided by your healthcare professional or as stated on the product label.

- Third, it should address temporary symptoms or conditions, not be a long-term solution.
- Fourth, regularly monitor your symptoms and overall progress while using sodium bicarbonate.
- Fifth, if your symptoms or condition persist, consider exploring alternative treatments or consulting your healthcare provider for other suitable options instead of relying solely on sodium bicarbonate.
- Sixth, address the root cause of your symptoms or condition rather than relying solely on sodium bicarbonate.
- Seventh, if using sodium bicarbonate for oral hygiene, limit its use and follow dental guidelines to prevent potential damage to tooth enamel.
- Eighth, do not consume excessive amounts of sodium bicarbonate.
- Finally, discard expired sodium bicarbonate products to prevent unintended usage beyond their shelf life.

Monitor sodium levels

Here are some tips to monitor sodium levels:

- First, consult a healthcare professional to assist you with the appropriate usage.
- Second, perform a baseline sodium level test to establish your initial sodium concentration.
- Third, follow your healthcare professional's recommendations for how often to conduct sodium level tests because regular testing helps monitor changes.
- Fourth, strictly adhere to the prescribed dosage of sodium bicarbonate.
- Fifth, drink adequate water to stay hydrated and maintain a balanced diet.
- Sixth, inform your healthcare provider about medications or supplements that might affect sodium levels.
- Seventh, regularly monitor your kidney function, as the kidneys

play an essential role in maintaining sodium levels in your body.
- Finally, familiarize yourself with the potential side effects of sodium bicarbonate that could affect sodium levels.

Dental precautions

- First, consult a dentist to assist you with the appropriate usage.
- Second, understand the specific dental purpose for using it, whether its teeth whitening, oral hygiene, or another dental concern.
- Third, if using baking soda toothpaste, use it in moderation.
- Fourth, continue with your regular dental hygiene routine, in addition to using sodium bicarbonate products.
- Fifth, brush your teeth using proper tooth-brushing techniques, including gentle circular motions and brushing for at least two minutes.

- Sixth, avoid aggressive or vigorous scrubbing of your teeth with baking soda toothpaste to prevent damage to tooth enamel.
- Seventh, regularly monitor the health of your gums and teeth.
- Eighth, consider alternating the use of baking soda toothpaste with your regular fluoride toothpaste to maintain the benefits of both.
- Ninth, after using a baking soda mouthwash or toothpaste, rinse your mouth thoroughly to remove any residue.
- Tenth, maintain regular dental check-ups to monitor your oral health and receive professional dental care.
- Finally, if using baking soda for teeth whitening, follow your dentist's recommendations to ensure safe and effective results.

Respiratory precautions

Here are tips for respiratory precautions:

- First, consult a respiratory therapist before using sodium bicarbonate for respiratory purposes.
- Second, adhere strictly to the recommended dosage and administration guidelines provided by your healthcare professional.
- Third, avoid self-medicating or using DIY treatments involving sodium bicarbonate for respiratory conditions without professional guidance.
- Fourth, administer sodium bicarbonate according to the frequency and duration specified by your healthcare professional.
- Fifth, monitor your respiratory symptoms carefully, including shortness of breath, coughing, and changes in sputum production. Report any significant changes to your healthcare provider.
- Sixth, use any aerosolized forms or nebulizer solutions as directed.
- Seventh, if using sodium bicarbonate with inhalation

devices like nebulizers, ensure the device is clean and in good working condition.
- Eighth, if you have existing respiratory conditions such as asthma, ensure that sodium bicarbonate use aligns with your overall respiratory management plan.
- Ninth, ensure adequate hydration during sodium bicarbonate use to help thin mucus and make it easier to expectorate.
- Finally, store sodium bicarbonate solutions properly, following storage guidelines provided by your healthcare professional or on the product label.

Adverse reactions

Here are some tips on how to handle adverse reactions:

- First, recognizing these symptoms is the first step in addressing adverse effects.
- Second, if sodium bicarbonate is ingested accidentally in a

significant amount, contact a poison control center.
- Third, if you experience gastrointestinal upset, stay well-hydrated to prevent dehydration. Drink plenty of water unless instructed otherwise by a healthcare professional.
- Fourth, do not mix sodium bicarbonate with acidic substances because it can cause gas and discomfort, aggravating adverse reactions.
- Fifth, allow yourself ample rest and monitor the symptoms carefully.
- Sixth, inform your healthcare provider about any adverse reactions you experience after using sodium bicarbonate. They can provide further guidance and recommend appropriate actions.
- Seventh, record the adverse reactions, including the time of occurrence, severity, duration, and any other relevant information that may assist your healthcare

provider in understanding the situation.
- Eighth, always follow the medical advice of your healthcare provider.
- Ninth, if you experience adverse reactions to sodium bicarbonate, discuss alternative solutions or treatments with your healthcare provider.
- Tenth, if adverse reactions are related to dosage, review the recommended dosage and ensure you are using the product correctly.

Child safety

Child safety when using sodium bicarbonate is essential to prevent accidental ingestion. Here are some important tips to help maintain a safe environment when using it around children:

- First, store sodium bicarbonate products, whether in powder or tablet form, in a secure,

childproof container, out of reach and sight of children.
- Second, store sodium bicarbonate products in childproof cabinets or drawers, ideally at higher levels where children cannot reach them.
- Third, teach children about sodium bicarbonate and emphasize that it's not meant for ingestion or play. Educate them on the importance of not consuming or handling it.
- Fourth, supervise children closely when using sodium bicarbonate, especially if they are involved in baking or cleaning activities where it's used.
- Fifth, avoid keeping sodium bicarbonate near play areas or toys to prevent accidental mixing or ingestion during play.
- Sixth, use child-friendly alternatives for baking or cleaning that do not resemble or contain harmful substances, making it less likely for children to mistake them for something edible.

- Seventh, be mindful of packaging and labeling to ensure it is not mistaken for food or consumed accidentally.
- Eighth, dispose of empty sodium bicarbonate containers to prevent accidental exposure or ingestion.
- Ninth, use child-safe cleaning products and ensure that sodium bicarbonate is not accessible to children during cleaning activities.
- Tenth, familiarize yourself and older children with basic first aid measures in case of accidental ingestion or exposure to sodium bicarbonate.
- Eleventh, keep emergency contact information, including the local poison control center, easily accessible in case of accidental ingestion or exposure.
- Twelfth, encourage safe practices around cleaning and baking.
- Thirteenth, schedule regular checkups with healthcare providers to ensure the child's

well-being and discuss household safety measures.
- Finally, be a role model by demonstrating safe handling and use of sodium bicarbonate, reinforcing responsible practices.

Storing safely

Here are some tips:

- First, clearly label the container with the contents to avoid confusion and accidental use.
- Second, store sodium bicarbonate in a location inaccessible to children, preferably in a high cabinet or pantry.
- Third, keep sodium bicarbonate away from household cleaning products, especially acidic ones, to prevent accidental mixing or reactions.
- Fourth, adhere to any specific storage instructions or guidelines provided on the packaging of the sodium bicarbonate product.

- Fifth, regularly check the expiration date on the packaging and dispose of any expired sodium bicarbonate. Replace it with a fresh supply.
- Sixth, store sodium bicarbonate away from strong-smelling items or substances to prevent the absorption of unwanted odors.
- Seventh, keep sodium bicarbonate separate from food items in the pantry to prevent accidental mix-ups.
- Eighth, avoid storing sodium bicarbonate near medications to prevent any mix-up or confusion.
- Twelfth, periodically inspect the container for signs of damage, leaks, or spoilage. Replace the container if needed.
- Finally, if storing a large quantity of sodium bicarbonate, consider dividing it into smaller, airtight containers to maintain freshness and quality.

Educating oneself

Here are some tips:

- First, explore credible websites, educational platforms, and scientific journals to learn about the properties, uses, and potential benefits of sodium bicarbonate.
- Second, consider attending workshops, classes, or seminars that pertain to baking, cooking, cleaning, or other practical applications where sodium bicarbonate is used.
- Third, enroll in online courses or webinars on chemistry, culinary arts, health, or cleaning and hygiene, where you can learn about the science and applications of sodium bicarbonate.
- Fourth, engage in online chemistry forums or communities to ask questions, share experiences, and learn from professionals or enthusiasts knowledgeable about sodium bicarbonate.

- Fifth, subscribe to scientific journals or magazines related to chemistry, health, or nutrition that publish research and articles about sodium bicarbonate.
- Sixth, follow reputable science channels, blogs, or YouTube channels that provide educational content on sodium bicarbonate, its properties, and applications.
- Seventh, attend talks or seminars organized by healthcare organizations, universities, or health centers to learn about the potential health benefits of sodium bicarbonate.
- Eighth, carefully read the labels and instructions on sodium bicarbonate products you purchase, understanding proper usage, dosage, and safety precautions.
- Ninth, safely conduct small experiments or activities using sodium bicarbonate at home, following appropriate guidelines and safety measures.

- Tenth, enroll in cooking or baking classes to learn firsthand about incorporating sodium bicarbonate into recipes and understanding its effects on cooking.
- Eleventh, keep yourself updated with the latest research and studies on sodium bicarbonate by regularly reviewing scientific publications and articles.
- Finally, maintain a curious mindset and seek to expand your knowledge and understanding of sodium bicarbonate and its applications through continuous learning.

Follow professional advice

Always follow the advice of healthcare professionals regarding the use of baking soda for specific health conditions.

- First, communicate your goals and concerns to the professional, whether your appointment is for medical, dental, or other purposes,

to help them provide tailored advice
- Second, adhere strictly to the recommended dosage and usage instructions provided by the healthcare professional.
- Third, update the healthcare professional about any changes in your health status while using sodium bicarbonate.
- Fourth, inform the professional about any other treatments, therapies, or alternative approaches you are taking in combination with sodium bicarbonate.
- Fifth, trust the expertise and guidance provided by the healthcare professional. Avoid self-adjusting dosage or altering the usage without consulting them.
- Sixth, if you have doubts about the advice received, seek a second opinion from another healthcare professional.
- Seventh, if sodium bicarbonate is used as part of a medical

treatment, follow the post-procedure instructions diligently for optimal results.
- Eighth, maintain open and honest communication with the healthcare professional throughout the process, providing updates on progress or any concerns.

- Ninth, if you experience positive outcomes or benefits from using sodium bicarbonate based on the professional's advice, share this information during follow-up appointments.

- Finally, continue to educate yourself about sodium bicarbonate and its applications, but always rely on professional advice for medical decisions.

CHAPTER EIGHT

APPLICATION TO VARIOUS CONDITIONS

Sodium bicarbonate has various applications in managing and alleviating different health conditions. This chapter highlights how it is used for several health conditions.

What is heartburn?

Heartburn is a type of discomfort in the chest. It feels like something hot or burning in the center of your chest. It occurs when the contents of your stomach enter your throat. This can happen after eating a lot or having some foods that can worsen.

Causes of heartburn

- Spicy, fatty, or acidic foods and beverages
- Excess weight, especially around the abdomen
- Hormonal changes and the pressure of the growing uterus can

lead to heartburn in pregnant individuals.

Symptoms of heartburn
- Burning sensation in the chest region
- Regurgitation
- Discomfort in the chest

How can you use baking soda to relief heartburn?
- First, consult your doctor.
- Second, ensure you have food-grade baking soda, water, a teaspoon for measuring, and a glass or cup for mixing.
- Third, measure half to one teaspoon of baking soda using a teaspoon.
- Fourth, mix the measured baking soda with a glass of water, about 5 ounces.
- Fifth, drink the baking soda mixture. It's usually best to drink it slowly to allow for better absorption and effectiveness.
- Sixth, allow some time for the baking soda to work.

- Seventh, follow the dosage instructions provided by your healthcare professional or on the packaging.
- Eighth, pay attention to how you feel after using the baking soda mixture.
- Ninth, use baking soda for heartburn only as an occasional, short-term remedy.
- Tenth, keep track of your sodium intake from all sources, including baking soda.

What is indigestion?

It is a frequent digestive condition of the upper digestive system. It is not an illness but a collection of symptoms that can arise from several reasons. Baking soda can provide temporary relief for indigestion symptoms by neutralizing stomach acid.

Causes of indigestion

- Eating spicy, fatty, or acidic foods that can irritate the digestive tract

- Emotional factors such as stress and anxiety can affect digestion and lead to indigestion.
- Excessive consumption of alcohol and caffeine
- Some medications can cause it.

Symptoms of indigestion

- Feeling full or bloated, even with a small amount of food
- Belching, flatulence, or an audible growling stomach
- Upper abdominal discomfort or pain

How can you use baking soda to relieve indigestion?
- First, consult a healthcare professional.
- Second, gather supplies and ensure you have food-grade baking soda, water, a teaspoon for measuring, and a glass or cup for mixing.
- Third, measure half to one teaspoon of baking soda using a teaspoon.

- Fourth, mix the measured baking soda with a glass of water, about 5 ounces.
- Fifth, drink the baking soda mixture. Drink it slowly for better absorption and effectiveness.
- Sixth, pay attention to how you feel after using the baking soda mixture. Monitor if your symptoms improve.
- Seventh, follow the dosage instructions provided by your healthcare professional or on the product packaging.
- Eighth, use baking soda for indigestion as an occasional, short-term remedy.
- Ninth, keep track of your sodium intake, as baking soda contains sodium. Excessive sodium can have health implications.
- Tenth, if you have persistent indigestion, consult a healthcare professional for appropriate evaluation and treatment.

What is metabolic acidosis?

It is a condition that happens when the body accumulates too much acid or loses too much base to balance the acid. This imbalance leads to increased acidity in the body, affecting normal functions and potentially causing various health issues.

Causes metabolic acidosis
- Impaired kidney function hampers the elimination of acids or the re-absorption of bicarbonate.
- Excessive loss of bicarbonate through the kidneys or gastrointestinal tract

Symptoms metabolic acidosis
- Rapid breathing
- Confusion or disorientation
- Fatigue and weakness
- Nausea and vomiting
- Headache
- Irregular heartbeat
- Muscle weakness or cramps
- Decreased appetite

How can you use baking soda to relieve metabolic acidosis?
- First, consult a healthcare provider.
- Second, allow the healthcare provider to guide the appropriate treatment, probably sodium bicarbonate, in a medical setting.
- Third, if your healthcare provider recommends using baking soda to relieve metabolic acidosis, they will administer it in a controlled and precise manner, often through intravenous injection.
- Fourth, follow your healthcare provider's recommendations.

What is dental plaque?

It is a type of biofilm that forms on the teeth and can cause several dental problems. It is a soft, sticky film of bacteria, food particles, and saliva that adheres to the teeth.

Causes of dental plaque
- Growth of bacteria in the mouth.
- Improper oral hygiene practices, such as infrequent brushing and

flossing, allow plaque to accumulate.

Symptoms of dental plaque
- White or pale yellow film on the teeth.
- The bacteria in dental plaque can produce foul-smelling compounds, leading to bad breath.
- Red, swollen, and bleeding gums.
- Eroding of the tooth enamel leads to cavities.
- Forms into tartar or calculus.

How can you use baking soda to treat dental plaque?

- First, mix a teaspoon of baking soda with water to make a paste.
- Second, wet your toothbrush with water.
- Third, dip the wet toothbrush into the baking soda paste.
- Fourth, gently brush your teeth with the baking soda paste in a circular motion for about two minutes.

- Fifth, rinse your mouth thoroughly with water to remove the baking soda residue.
- Sixth, spit out any remaining residue.
- Seventh, after using the baking soda paste, brush your teeth with your regular fluoride toothpaste to ensure all areas are cleaned and benefit from fluoride.
- Eighth, use this baking soda paste once or twice a week, not more frequently, to avoid potential enamel erosion due to its abrasive nature.
- Ninth, always consult your dentist before using baking soda to ensure it is safe for you to use for your oral health.

What is eczema?

Eczema is a common skin condition characterized by red, itchy, and inflamed patches. It's not contagious and usually involves periods of flare-ups and periods of improvement.

Causes of eczema
- Overactive immune responses to irritants and allergens lead to skin inflammation.
- Exposure to irritants such as soaps, detergents, certain fabrics, allergens, and extreme weather conditions
- Compromised skin barrier
- Food allergies, such as "dairy, eggs, and nuts, cause flare-ups.

Symptoms of eczema
- Itching is the characteristic symptom of eczema and can be intense, leading to scratching and further skin damage.
- Affected skin areas are often red.
- Eczema patches may have scales or small, raised bumps.
- Affected areas may become swollen.
- Ooze clear or yellowish fluid and develop crusts.
- Constant scratching
- Changes in skin pigmentation.

- Constant scratching and broken skin can lead to secondary bacterial or viral skin infections.

How can you use baking soda to relieve eczema symptoms?

- First, mix two tablespoons of baking soda with water to create a thick yet spreadable paste.
- Second, test a small amount of the paste on a small area to check for adverse reactions or skin sensitivity.
- Third, gently apply the baking soda paste to the affected areas of the skin with eczema.
- Fourth, leave the paste on for a short period of 12 minutes.
- Fifth, after the designated time, gently rinse the baking soda paste off with warm water.
- Sixth, gently pat the skin dry before applying a moisturizer to lock in moisture.
- Seventh, only use this baking soda paste once a week to avoid skin irritation.

- Eighth, if you have severe eczema or persistent symptoms, consult a dermatologist or a healthcare professional for personalized advice and treatment options.

What is foot odor?

Foot odor is an unpleasant odor caused by sweat interacting with bacteria on the skin, breaking it down and producing an unpleasant odor.

Causes of foot odor
- Excessive sweating leads to a moist environment in which odor-causing bacteria survive.
- Bacteria present on the skin break down sweat, producing an unpleasant odor.
- Wearing tight or poorly ventilated shoes and socks can trap moisture, fostering the growth of bacteria and fungi.
- Emotional stress can lead to excessive sweating and exacerbating foot odor.

Symptoms of foot odor
- A distinctive, foul smell emitted from the feet is the primary symptom.
- Feet may feel persistently moist due to excessive sweating.

How can you use baking soda to manage foot odor
- First, fill a basin halfway with warm water and stir in a few tablespoons of baking soda.
- Second, soak your feet for 20 minutes and pat your feet dry thoroughly.
- Third, after drying your feet, put baking soda directly into your shoes or socks to absorb moisture and neutralize odors.
- Fourth, create a paste using a small amount of water and baking soda. Gently scrub the paste onto your feet, focusing on areas prone to odor.
- Fifth, rinse thoroughly and dry your feet.

What are mouth ulcers?

They are small, painful lesions that develop on the soft tissues inside the mouth.

Causes of mouth ulcers
- Injury to the mouth
- Nutritional deficiencies
- Immune system issues
- Viral/bacterial infections

Symptoms of mouth ulcers
- Painful sores
- Discomfort while eating, drinking, or speaking.

How can you use baking soda to alleviate mouth ulcers?
- First, mix a teaspoon of baking soda with water to make the rinse.
- Second, rinse your mouth by taking a mouthful of the solution.
- Third, swish the mixture around your mouth for about 45 seconds.
- Fourth, spit out the solution and rinse your mouth with plain water.
- Fifth, repeat as needed by rinsing three times a day.

What is sunburned skin?

Sunburned skin is the red, painful, and sometimes swollen skin that happens when you stay in the sun for too long without proper protection. It causes skin redness, warmth, and sometimes blistering.

Causes of sunburned skin
- Prolonged exposure to UV radiation which damages the skin
- Factors such as the intensity of the sun, the duration of exposure, and the skin's sensitivity to UV rays can influence the severity.

Symptoms of sunburned skin
- Redness of affected area and may feel warm to the touch.
- Sunburned skin is often painful and tender
- Swelling and blisters
- Peeling skin

How can you use baking soda to offer relief for sunburn skin?
- First, dissolve half a cup of baking soda in the bath water.

- Second, stir the water to help the baking soda dissolve.
- Third, soak in the baking soda bath for about 20 minutes.
- Fourth, gently pat your skin dry with a soft towel to prevent further irritation.
- Fifth, avoid using hot water because it can aggravate sunburned skin.

What are chemical burns?

Chemical burns are skin and underlying tissue injuries caused by chemical contact. Acids, alkalis, solvents, or other hazardous chemicals can cause these burns.

Causes of chemical burns
- Direct contact of skin with a corrosive chemical
- Accidental splashes, spills, or splatters of chemicals can lead to chemical burns.

Symptoms of chemical burns
- The affected skin areas often become reddish
- Pain in the affected area

- Blisters may form on the skin
- It can lead to the development of ulcers or open sores

How can you use baking soda to provide relief to chemical burns?

- First, immediately rinse the affected area with cool running water to flush out the chemicals and help reduce the extent of the burn.
- Second, gently remove clothing or jewelry near the affected area to ensure no chemicals remain on the skin.
- Third, make a baking soda paste by combining three parts baking soda and one part water.
- Fourth, gently apply the baking soda paste to the affected area, covering the burn with a thin layer.
- Fifth, leave the paste on for a short duration of approximately 20 minutes.
- Sixth, after the designated time, rinse the area gently with cool

water to remove the baking soda paste.
- Seventh, if needed, you can repeat the baking soda paste application a few times daily for comfort.
- Eighth, if the burn is extensive and the pain is severe, seek medical help immediately.

What are insect bites or stings?

Insect bites or stings are injuries caused by bugs such as "mosquitoes, bees, or ants."

Causes of insect bites or stings
- Mosquitoes bite to feed on blood, and their saliva can cause localized skin irritation and itching.
- Bees and wasps sting in self-defense when they feel threatened. They inject venom through their stingers.
- Fire ants can deliver painful bites with venomous stings.

- Some spider species can deliver bites that may result in localized skin reactions.
- Bedbugs feed on human blood and can cause itchy, red, and raised skin lesions.

Symptoms of insect bites or stings
- The affected area may become swollen, red, or inflamed.
- Itching
- The skin around the bite or sting site may become red.
- It can result in a rash
- It can result in fluid-filled blisters
- Scratching can introduce bacteria and lead to infections.
- Difficulty breathing hives
- Swelling of the face and throat

How can you use baking soda to provide relief to insect bites or stings?
- First, baking soda paste should be prepared by mixing baking soda with water.

- Second, gently clean the area around the insect bite or sting with mild soap and water.
- Third, apply the baking soda paste directly to the affected area of the insect bite or sting.
- Fourth, leave the paste on for approximately 20 minutes to allow it to provide relief from itching and irritation.
- Fifth, gently rinse off the baking soda paste with cool water.
- Sixth, pat the area dry with a clean towel.
- Seventh, if the itching persists, you can reapply the baking soda paste as needed, following the same steps.
- Eighth, if you experience severe reactions, allergic symptoms, or the bite appears infected, seek medical attention immediately.

What is a poison oak rash?

A poison oak rash is a skin reaction caused by contact with the native North American poison oak plant (Toxicodendron diversilobum). The rash results from exposure to urushiol, the oil found in poison oak, poison ivy, and poison sumac. When urushiol comes into contact with the skin, it can cause an itchy and often uncomfortable rash.

Causes of poison oak rash
- Direct or indirect contact with urushiol, the allergenic oil found in poison oak leaves, stems, and roots.
- Touching poison oak plants, including leaves, stems, or roots can transfer urushiol to the skin.

Symptoms of poison oak rash
- Itchy skin is one of the symptoms of a poison oak rash.
- The affected skin often becomes red and inflamed.
- The rash can be painful, especially if the blisters burst or become infected.
- In severe cases, the rash may weep clear or yellowish fluid and develop crusts.
- Symptoms typically appear within 20 to 70 hours.

How can you use baking soda to provide relief to poison oak rash?

- First, baking soda paste should be prepared by mixing baking soda with water.
- Second, gently clean the area around the insect bite or sting with mild soap and water.
- Third, apply the baking soda paste to the affected area, covering the poison oak rash with a thin layer.
- Fourth, allow the baking soda paste to sit on the rash for approximately 20 minutes.
- Fifth, after the designated time, rinse the area gently with cool water to remove the baking soda paste.
- Sixth, repeat the baking soda paste application two times daily for comfort.
- Seventh, if the rash is severe and you experience difficulty breathing or a fever, seek medical attention immediately.

What is optimal exercise performance?

Exercise performance is how good you are at engaging in running or playing sports by giving you extra energy to do your best.

Factors affecting exercise performance

- Fitness level
- Training and conditioning
- Nutrition
- Hydration
- Rest and recovery
- Psychological factors
- Genetics
- Equipment and gear
- Environmental conditions

Symptoms of optimal exercise performance

- Increased stamina and the ability to sustain physical effort over extended periods
- Enhanced muscular strength, which enables lifting heavier weights or performing more challenging exercises

- Improved speed and agility, leading to faster running, jumping, and other movements
- Decreased feelings of fatigue during and after exercise
- Improved mental focus, concentration, and determination during physical activities
- A boost in mood and reduced stress and anxiety were due to the release of endorphins during exercise.
- Better weight control and body composition

How can you use baking soda to boost exercise performance?

- First, consult with a healthcare professional.
- Second, work with a healthcare provider to determine the appropriate dosage of it.
- Third, before exercising, consume it over several days to improve its effects. This involves consuming small doses-for instance, 0.3 grams per kg of body weight

spread throughout the day for 4 days before exercise.
- Fourth, observe how your body reacts to the baking soda. Some individuals may experience gastrointestinal discomfort, so it's essential to monitor tolerance and adjust the dosage if needed.
- Fifth, drink plenty of water throughout the day.
- Sixth, monitor your exercise performance, endurance, and perceived fatigue to determine if baking soda has any positive effects.
- Seventh, assess whether the use of baking soda positively impacts your exercise performance.

What are kidney diseases?

A kidney disease is a medical condition that affects the kidneys' structure and function.

Causes of kidney diseases
- Prolonged high blood pressure.
- Unrestrained diabetes

- Untreated bacterial or viral infections
- Autoimmune diseases
- Medications and toxins
- Physical injuries or trauma to the kidneys can cause acute kidney injury

Symptoms of kidney diseases
- Persistent fatigue and weakness
- Edema, the accumulation of fluid in the body, often leads to swelling in the legs, ankles, face, and abdomen.
- Alterations in urine output, color, or frequency
- Blood in the urine
- High blood pressure
- Kidney pain or discomfort in the lower
- Nausea and vomiting
- Severe itching due to the buildup of toxins in the body
- Difficulty breathing can result from fluid retention and pulmonary edema.
- Weakened bones and bone pain may occur due to imbalances in

minerals like calcium and phosphorus.

How can you use baking soda to prevent kidney diseases?

- First, consult with a healthcare provider.
- Second, talk to your healthcare provider about using baking soda as a potential preventive measure for kidney diseases or to manage conditions like metabolic acidosis.
- Third, collaborate with your doctor to determine the proper dosage.
- Fourth, if baking soda is recommended, your healthcare provider will likely establish a schedule for monitoring your kidney function and adjusting the dosage as needed.
- Fifth, adhere to the dosage and administration recommendations provided by your healthcare provider.
- Sixth, maintain a balanced diet and stay well-hydrated to support overall kidney health.

- Seventh, engage in regular physical activity to help support kidney health.
- Eighth, attend regular check-ups with your healthcare provider to monitor your kidney function and overall health.

Baking soda and pets

It is used to treat some health issues in pets, but it must be used safely and in appropriate dosages. However, before giving any substance to your pet, always consult a veterinarian.

Uses and considerations for pets

- It can be used in your pet's bedding.
- It can be used in oral health as an ingredient in homemade toothpaste for pets.
- It can be used as part of a natural flea bath for pets.
- It can be used as a dry shampoo for pets, especially cats, who may not tolerate traditional baths.

- It can help relieve itching and discomfort from insect bites and stings in pets.

What is oral hygiene for pets?

Oral hygiene for pets entails caring for and maintaining their dental health to avoid dental issues such as periodontal disease, tooth decay, and bad breath. It includes practices to maintain clean teeth, healthy gums, and a fresh mouth. Good oral hygiene for pets typically involves regular brushing, veterinary check-ups, a proper diet, dental chews or toys, professional cleanings, and monitoring oral health.

How can you use baking soda for oral hygiene in pets?

- First, create a baking soda paste by mixing it with water.
- Second, brush your pet's teeth gently using a soft toothbrush.
- Third, ensure your pet tolerates the taste and the brushing process.
- Fourth, dilute baking soda in water to create a gentle oral rinse.

- Fifth, use a cotton swab or gauze to wipe your pet's gums and teeth with the solution.

What is odor in pet's bedding?

Odor in a pet's bedding refers to an unpleasant smell that emanates from the fabric or material used in the bedding due to various factors such as accumulated body oils and saliva, residual urine or feces, bacterial growth, dust, dirt, and dander.

How can you use baking soda to control the odor in your pet's bedding?

- First, prepare the bedding by removing the bedding from the pet's area.
- Second, lightly sprinkle baking soda over the surface of the bedding for 20 minutes.
- Third, shake and beat it outdoors to remove the baking soda.

- Fourth, allow the bedding to air in the sun to eliminate odors.

What are the itching and discomfort from insect bites and stings in pets?

Itching and discomfort from insect bites and stings in pets can vary depending on the animal's sensitivity and the type of insect.

Symptoms

- Localized redness
- Pets may frequently scratch or bite at the affected area.
- Pets show signs of discomfort or pain
- Swelling and inflammation may be visible at the bite site
- Pets may paw at or lick the affected area in an attempt to alleviate discomfort
- Restlessness could be observed if the irritation is substantial

- Symptoms might include hives, difficulty breathing, or more pronounced swelling.

How can you use baking soda to offer relief for it in pets?

- Baking soda can aid in relieving itching and discomfort from insect bites or stings in pets.
- First, create a baking soda paste by mixing it with water.
- Second, gently apply the paste to the affected area where the pet was bitten or stung, and ensure the paste covers the irritated skin.
- Third, leave the paste on for about 15 minutes.
- Fourth, gently rinse the area with lukewarm water to remove the baking soda paste.
- Fifth, pat the area dry with a clean towel.

CHAPTER NINE

CONCLUSIONS

- It has highlighted the complete, step-by-step guide on how baking soda treats various health conditions, prevents kidney diseases, applies to pets, and boosts exercise performance.
- It has highlighted the chemistry of sodium bicarbonate, including its composition, reactions, and applications in baking, cleaning, and medicine.
- It has also highlighted several healing actions and properties due to its alkaline properties and ability to neutralize acids.
- It has highlighted the devices used with sodium bicarbonate for administering it to different health conditions.
- It has also highlighted ways baking soda can be consumed in various ways, depending on the intended use.
- It has also highlighted several precautions to be taken when

using baking soda to treat different health challenges to ensure its safe and effective use.
- It has highlighted the applications in managing and alleviating different health conditions, both in humans and pets.

Index

Abrasive properties, 51
Acid-base properties, 26
Adverse reactions, 95
Agricultural grade, 40
Alkaline properties, 53
alkaline substances, 19
Alkalinity, 28
Alkalization properties, 54
Antacid properties, 51
Antacid tablets, 81
Antifungal, 53
Anti-inflammatory, 52
APPLICATION TO VARIOUS CONDITIONS, 107
Avoid prolonged use, 89
baking soda, 14
Baking soda and pets, 134
Baking soda paste, 76
Baking soda solution, 75
Benefits, 18
Beverage additive, 83
Bicarbonate ion, 25
Buffering capacity, 55
chemical burns, 122
Chemical industries, 30
Chemical properties, 44
Chemical structure, 25
CHEMISTRY OF SODIUM BICARBONATE, 25
Child safety, 97
Commercial suppliers, 31
CONCLUSIONS, 139
Consulting healthcare professional, 85
contemporary times, 23
Cooking and baking, 77
Cosmetic grade, 41
crystallization, 35
Decomposition, 28
Dental applications, 64
dental plaque, 113
Dental precautions, 92
DEVICES, 56
Dissolved in juice, 84
Dosage and administration, 87
eczema, 115
Educating oneself, 102
Electrolysis, 34
Extraction Methods, 31
Follow professional advice, 104
Food grade, 36
foot odor, 118
Gastrointestinal tubes, 61
Grades, 36
HEALING ACTIONS, 51
healing with baking, 15
heartburn, 107
HISTORY, 19
indigestion, 109
Industrial grade, 39
Infusion pumps, 67
insect bites, 124
Intravenous administration devices, 58
INTRODUCTION, 12

kidney diseases, 131
Laboratory preparation, 46
Leavening, 20
Leavening action, 27
medicinal use, 21
metabolic acidosis, 112
Mining, 31
Mining and extraction, 30
Monitor sodium levels, 91
mouth ulcers, 120
mouthwash dispenser, 65
Myths, 17
Natural deposits, 29
Nebulizers, 56
Neutralization reaction, 33
odor in pet's bedding, 136
odor-neutralizing properties, 53
optimal exercise performance, 129
oral conditions, 72
oral hygiene for pets, 135
Oral rinse, 79
pH regulation, 28
Pharmaceutical grade, 37
Pharmacopeia grade, 37
Physical properties, 42
poison oak rash, 126
PRECAUTIONS, 85
production era, 21

PROPERTIES, 51
Pros and cons, 15
Purification, 35
Reaction with acids, 27
Reaction with carbon dioxide, 33
Reagent grade, 40
recovery of sodium carbonate, 49
regeneration of ammonium chloride, 49
Respiratory precautions, 93
Retail stores, 31
Skin and scalp applicators, 70
Solution mining, 32
Solvay process, 33
soothing properties, 52
Specialty grades, 42
Sprayers, 72
stings, 124
stings in pets, 137
Storing safely, 100
sunburned skin, 121
Supplements, 82
Synthetic production, 29
Technical grade, 38
The commercial production, 47
toothbrush for oral hygiene, 64
Toothpaste, 80
urinary alkalinization, 67
Uses and considerations for pets, 134